certain other noncommercial uses

permitted by copyright law

Contents

Why Dieting Is Important

The importance of dieting cannot be overstated. Eating healthy foods is essential for good health and proper nutrition. A balanced diet that includes nutritious, whole foods provides the body with the fuel it needs to function optimally. Eating unhealthy foods, on the other hand, can lead to health problems, including obesity, heart disease, diabetes, and other chronic illnesses.

When it comes to dieting, the goal is to eat the right kinds of foods in the right amounts to maintain a healthy weight. Eating a balanced diet with plenty of fruits, vegetables, whole grains, lean proteins, and healthy fats can help ensure that you get the vitamins, minerals, and other nutrients your body needs. Eating a variety of foods also helps to ensure that you get all of the essential nutrients your body needs.

The benefits of dieting go beyond just maintaining a healthy weight. Eating a nutritious, balanced diet can also help to reduce the risk of developing certain chronic diseases. Eating a diet rich in fruits and vegetables, for example, can reduce the risk of developing certain types of cancer. Eating a diet high in fiber-rich foods can lower cholesterol levels and reduce the risk of heart disease. Eating a diet low in saturated fats and high in unsaturated fats can help to lower blood pressure and reduce the risk of stroke.

Eating a healthy diet can also help to improve mental health. Eating a diet rich in fruits and vegetables, for example, can help to improve mood and increase energy levels. Eating a diet high in healthy fats, such as those found in fish, can help to reduce anxiety and improve cognitive performance.

Finally, dieting is important for overall health. Eating a nutritious, balanced diet can help to reduce the risk of developing certain chronic diseases, improve mental health, and improve overall well-being. Eating a healthy diet can also help to reduce the risk of obesity, which can increase the risk of developing certain types of cancer and other chronic illnesses.

In short, dieting is an essential part of maintaining good health. Eating a nutritious, balanced diet can help to reduce the risk of developing certain chronic diseases, improve mental health, and improve overall well-being. Eating a healthy diet can also help to reduce the risk of obesity, which can increase the risk of developing certain types of cancer and other chronic illnesses. For these reasons, it is important to make sure that you are eating a nutritious, balanced diet that includes plenty of fruits and vegetables, whole grains, lean proteins, and healthy fats.

What Causes Chronic Pain?

Overview

Everyone experiences occasional aches and pains. In fact, sudden pain is an important reaction of the nervous system that helps alert you to possible injury. When an injury occurs, pain signals travel from the injured area up your spinal cord and to your brain.

Pain will usually become less severe as the injury heals. However, chronic pain is different from typical pain. With chronic pain, your body continues to send pain signals to your brain, even after an injury heals. This can last several weeks to years. Chronic pain can limit your mobility and reduce your flexibility, strength, and endurance. This may make it challenging to get through daily tasks and activities.

Chronic pain is defined as pain that lasts at least 12 weeks. The pain may feel sharp or dull, causing a burning or aching sensation in the affected areas. It may be steady or intermittent, coming and going without any apparent reason. Chronic pain can occur in nearly any part of your body. The pain can feel different in the various affected areas.

Some of the most common types of chronic pain include:

- headache

- postsurgical pain

- post-trauma pain

- lower back pain

- cancer pain

- arthritis pain

- neurogenic pain (pain caused by nerve damage)

- psychogenic pain (pain that isn't caused by disease, injury, or nerve damage)

According to the American Academy of Pain Medicine, more than 1.5 billion people around the world have chronic pain. It's the most common cause of long-term disability in the United States, affecting about 100 million Americans.

What causes chronic pain?

Chronic pain is usually caused by an initial injury, such as a back sprain or pulled muscle. It's believed that chronic pain develops after nerves become damaged. The nerve damage makes pain more intense and long lasting. In these cases, treating the underlying injury may not resolve the chronic pain.

In some cases, however, people experience chronic pain without any prior injury. The exact causes of chronic pain without injury aren't well understood. The pain may sometimes result from an underlying health condition, such as:

• chronic fatigue syndrome: characterized by extreme, prolonged weariness that's often accompanied by pain

• endometriosis: a painful disorder that occurs when the uterine lining grows outside of the uterus

- fibromyalgia: widespread pain in the bones and muscles

- inflammatory bowel disease: a group of conditions that causes painful, chronic inflammation in the digestive tract

- interstitial cystitis: a chronic disorder marked by bladder pressure and pain

- temporomandibular joint dysfunction (TMJ): a condition that causes painful clicking, popping, or locking of the jaw

- vulvodynia: chronic vulva pain that occurs with no obvious cause

Who is at risk for chronic pain?

Chronic pain can affect people of all ages, but it's most common in older adults. Besides age, other factors that can increase your risk of developing chronic pain include:

- having an injury

- having surgery

- being female

- being overweight or obese

How is chronic pain treated?

The main goal of treatment is to reduce pain and boost mobility. This helps you return to your daily activities without discomfort.

The severity and frequency of chronic pain can differ among individuals. So doctors create pain management plans that are specific to each person. Your pain management plan will depend on your symptoms and any underlying health conditions. Medical treatments, lifestyle remedies, or a combination of these methods may be used to treat your chronic pain.

Medications for chronic pain

Several types of medications are available that can help treat chronic pain. Here are a few examples:

- over-the-counter pain relievers, including acetaminophen (Tylenol) or nonsteroidal anti-inflammatory drugs (NSAIDs) such as aspirin (Bufferin) or ibuprofen (Advil).

- opioid pain relievers, including morphine (MS Contin), codeine, and hydrocodone (Tussigon)

- adjuvant analgesics, such as antidepressants and anticonvulsants

Medical procedures for chronic pain

Certain medical procedures can also provide relief from chronic pain. An example of a few are:

- electrical stimulation, which reduces pain by sending mild electric shocks into your muscles

- nerve block, which is an injection that prevents nerves from sending pain signals to your brain

- acupuncture, which involves lightly pricking your skin with needles to alleviate pain

- surgery, which corrects injuries that may have healed improperly and that may be contributing to the pain

Lifestyle remedies for chronic pain

Additionally, various lifestyle remedies are available to help ease chronic pain. Examples include:

- physical therapy

- tai chi

- yoga

- art and music therapy

- pet therapy

- psychotherapy

- massage

* meditation

Dealing with chronic pain

There isn't a cure for chronic pain, but the condition can be managed successfully. It's important to stick to your pain management plan to help relieve symptoms.

Physical pain is related to emotional pain, so chronic pain can increase your stress levels. Building emotional skills can help you cope with any stress related to your condition. Here are some steps you can take to reduce stress:

Take good care of your body: Eating well, getting enough sleep, and exercising regularly can keep your body healthy and reduce feelings of stress.

Continue taking part in your daily activities: You can boost your mood and decrease stress by participating in activities you enjoy and socializing with friends. Chronic pain may make it challenging to perform certain tasks. But isolating yourself can give you a more negative outlook on your condition and increase your sensitivity to pain.

Seek support: Friends, family, and support groups can lend you a helping hand and offer comfort during difficult times. Whether you're having trouble with daily tasks or you're simply in need of an emotional boost, a close friend or loved one can provide the support you need.

For more information and resources, visit the American Chronic Pain Association website at theacpa.org.

Banting Diet: Does It Work for Weight Loss?

The Banting diet dates back to 1862 and was touted as an almost miraculous way to treat obesity. Although slightly modified, it regained popularity in 2013 as a low carb, high fat (LCHF) way of eating.

The diet limits the intake of carbs almost entirely. It also promises to revert type 2 diabetes and high blood pressure, as well as improve your energy levels and sleep quality — all while causing drastic weight loss.

For some, the Banting diet becomes a way of life, but for others, limiting their carb intake is far too restrictive and unsustainable in the long term.

This article reviews the pros and cons of the Banting diet and tells you whether it works for weight loss.

BOTTOM LINE: The Banting diet eliminates one food group almost entirely. However, it encourages eating wholesome foods over processed ones, and its multiple communities may provide the needed support to sustain the diet in the long run.

What is the Banting diet?

The Banting diet was first prescribed to William Banting in 1862 by Dr. William Harvey as a weight loss diet.

William Banting's success with the diet led him to write a booklet that popularized the low carb strategy for weight loss, to the extent that the word "banting" became the name of the method, as well as a verb.

Recently, Tim Noakes, a South African scientist and professor, brought the method back into the spotlight after trying the Banting diet himself and writing the book

"Real Meal Revolution." His take on the diet is referred to as Banting 2.0.

The original Banting diet included four daily meals, which mainly comprised protein and restricted carbs — 1 ounce (30 grams) of dry bread in every meal and 2–3 ounces (60–90 grams) of fruit as a snack. It restricted bread, beans, butter, milk, sugar, beer, and potatoes.

However, Tim Noakes' approach is slightly different.

Banting 2.0 divides the process into four phases — observation, restoration, transformation, and preservation — and offers multiple food lists and structured meal plans to simplify the low carb approach.

It still restricts carbs to some extent, and its macronutrient composition resembles the keto diet with less than 5–10% of your daily calories coming from carbs, 65–90% from fat, and 10–35% from protein.

Still, both versions of the diet promise extreme weight loss, higher energy levels, improved sleep quality, reduced feelings of hunger, and increased feelings of overall well-being.

This article focuses on Noakes' newer version of the Banting diet.

SUMMARY

The Banting diet is a low carb, high fat diet that's very similar to the keto diet. It claims to improve energy levels, sleep, and overall well-being while causing weight loss.

How to follow the Banting diet

The Banting diet is divided into four phases that are meant to ease the transition into a LCHF way of life.

While you may follow the diet on your own, there's an online course available for those who want to dive into it with a structured and personalized Banting meal plan.

The course offers a step-by-step guide, recipes, optional daily support from a coach, and weekly mindset workshops to help manage temptations and make the transition smoother.

Phase 1: Observation

During this 1-week phase, you're supposed to follow your current diet without making any modifications.

It encourages you to track and journal everything you eat to figure out how you respond to food.

Phase 2: Restoration

The restoration phase is meant to restore your gut health and get you used to the Banting way of eating.

This phase may last 2–12 weeks, depending on your weight loss goal. Overall, you should follow it for 1 week for every 11 pounds (5 kg) of weight you want to lose.

During this time, you'll be introduced to a series of food lists. You're meant to eliminate all foods from the Red and Light Red lists and instead rely on those on the Green and Orange lists.

One plus is that there's no calorie counting or portion control in this phase.

Phase 3: Transformation

The transformation phase introduces you to the original Banting diet.

It takes your newly developed eating habits and cuts your carb intake to achieve ketosis, which is meant to get you into a rapid fat-burning mode.

To make this possible, the method encourages you to stick to foods on the Green list, while adding those on the Orange list to the no-go foods — along with the Red lists mentioned before.

This third phase lasts as long as it takes you to reach your desired weight, and you should track your meals for a couple of days every two weeks.

Additionally, the phase includes "lifestyle hacks," such as intermittent fasting, exercise tips, and sleep and meditation to avoid reaching a weight loss plateau.

The transformation phase is supposed to improve mental clarity, sleep, acne, and skin irritations, as well as even eradicate joint pain.

Phase 4: Preservation

This final phase, which is supposed to last indefinitely, starts once you've reached your desired weight. It's meant to help you maintain your new weight in the long run.

This is a more flexible phase, as you'll be able to reintroduce foods that are not allowed in the previous phase. The goal is to determine which ones you can safely eat without gaining weight.

Again, there's no food tracking during this phase, and you may follow the food lists as follows:

• Green: no limitations

- Orange: eat in moderation

- Light Red: hardly ever or on special occasions

- Red: never

- Gray: it's up to you

You can always return to the previous phase if you feel like you have lost control of your weight.

The Banting diet is divided into four phases, but ultimately it's meant to guide you into a new way of life. You start making changes in the second and third phases, and the fourth one allows a little flexibility.

Foods to eat and avoid

The Banting diet provides multiple food lists to eat and avoid.

Green list

This list includes foods that you may eat without restriction.

- Fruits and vegetables: leafy green vegetables, artichoke hearts, aubergine, asparagus, bean and Brussels sprouts, broccoli, green beans, cabbage, cauliflower, celery, chard, courgettes, cucumber, endive, fennel, garlic, germ squash, kale, leeks, lemon and lime, lettuce, mange tout, mushrooms, olives, onions, okra, palm hearts, peppers, radicchio, radishes, rhubarb, rocket, shallots, spinach, spring onions, snap peas, tomatoes, and turnips

• Meat, fish, and poultry: all meat, poultry, fish, seafood, offal, and naturally cured meats (i.e., pancetta, salami, parma ham, bacon, jerky, coppa (capocollo), and biltong), eggs, homemade bone broth, and cheeses, such as Brie, Camembert, Gorgonzola, Roquefort, mozzarella, feta, ricotta, Cheddar, Gouda, Emmental, Parmesan, and pecorino

- Drinks: caffeine-free herbal teas, flavored waters, and plain water

- Condiments: all kinds of vinegar and fermented soy sauce or tamari

- Fermented foods: coconut yogurt and kefir, kefir butter and cheese, kimchi, milk kefir, naturally fermented pickles, and sauerkraut

- Fats: any rendered animal fat, avocado, butter, ghee, cream, coconut oil, fruit and nut oils, mayonnaise, and seeds

Orange list

According to the method, foods on the Orange list offer multiple health benefits but may hinder your weight loss journey if consumed without restriction. Thus, foods on this list are meant to be enjoyed in moderation.

• Nuts: all raw nuts and sugar-free nut butters

• Dairy: milk and milk substitutes, cottage and cream cheese, full fat yogurt, and sour cream

• Fruits: apples, apricots, bananas, blueberries, blackberries, cherries, clementines, fresh figs, gooseberries, granadilla, grapes, guava, jackfruit, kiwi, kumquats, litchis, loquats, mangoes, nectarines, orange, papaya, pears, peaches, persimmon, pineapple, plantain, plums, pomegranates, quinces, raspberries, starfruit, strawberries, tangerines, tamarind pulp, and watermelon

• Drinks: caffeinated tea and coffee

• Legumes and pulses: all legumes, alfalfa, beans, chickpeas, and lentils

• Fermented foods: water kefir and kombucha

• Fruits and vegetables: beetroot, butternut squash, baby corn, carrots, calabash, cassava, celeriac, corn, edamame, golden beets, Hubbard squash, jicama, parsnips, peas, potatoes, pumpkins, rutabagas, spaghetti squash, and sweet potatoes

Light Red list

You should hardly ever consume foods on this list.

• Smoothies and vegetable juices: fruit and yogurt smoothies without frozen yogurt or ice cream, as well as vegetable juices without added fruit juice

- Treats and chocolate: dark chocolate (80% and above), dried fruit, honey, and pure maple syrup

- Gluten-free grains: amaranth, arrowroot, buckwheat, bran, gluten-free pasta, millet, oats, popcorn, quinoa, rice, sorghum, quinoa, tapioca, and teff

- Flours: almond, coconut, corn, chickpea, pea, and rice flours, polenta, and maize meal

Red list

This is probably the most important list, as it includes the foods you should never eat.

- General foods: fast food, foods with added sugar, chips, and sugary condiments, such as ketchup, dressings, and marinades

- Sweets: all confectionery and non-dark chocolates, artificial sweeteners, agave, canned fruit, coconut sugar, cordials, fructose, glucose, jam, malt, rice malt syrup, sugar, and golden syrup

- Gluten: barley, bulgur, couscous, durum, einkorn, farina, graham flour, Khorasan wheat (kamut), matzo, orzo, rye, semolina, spelt, triticale, wheat, and wheat germ

- Grain-based products: all commercial breaded or battered foods, breakfast cereals, and all crackers

- Drinks: energy drinks, soft drinks, commercial juices, commercial iced teas, flavored milks, and milkshakes

- Dairy-related foods: coffee creamers, commercial cheese spreads, condensed milk, ice cream, and commercial frozen yogurt

- Fats: butter spreads, canola oil, corn oil, cottonseed oil, margarine and shortening, rice bran oil, and sunflower and safflower oil

- Processed meats: highly processed sausages and meats cured with sugar

Gray list

The Gray list contains foods that fit the Banting diet but would slow your progress, so they're left to your discretion.

- Treats: Banting baked goods and sugar-free ice cream

- Sweeteners: xylitol, erythritol, isomalt, stevia powder, and sucralose

- Drinks: all alcoholic beverages, protein shakes, and supplements

- Vegetarian proteins: naturally fermented tofu, pea protein, and processed soy

SUMMARY

The Banting diet encourages you to avoid highly processed foods and opt for wholesome ones instead. It also limits gluten, high sugar foods, starches, dairy, and caffeine.

Is it effective for weight loss?

While there's no research on the Banting diet itself, there's plenty of scientific evidence supporting the LCHF approach for weight loss.

When restricting carbs, the body is stimulated to maximize fat oxidation to meet energy demands. This means that LCHF diets rely primarily on fats to produce energy (3Trusted Source).

Research suggests that there may be two different mechanisms behind the LCHF diet's success — increased feelings of fullness and a specific metabolic advantage.

Studies show people on LCHF diets given unrestricted access to foods don't necessarily consume more calories than people on low fat, high carb (LFHC) diets because they tend to perceive less hunger, and thus, reduce their overall food intake.

Additionally, LCHF diets usually lead to a higher protein intake, which also promotes feelings of fullness, and fewer cases of rebound hypoglycemia or low blood sugar levels, a common cause of hunger in those following high carb diets.

Regarding the alleged metabolic advantage, scientists attribute it to either an increased thermogenic effect from the protein intake, a higher protein turnover for gluconeogenesis, or loss of energy through the excretion of ketones in sweat or urine.

The thermogenic effect of foods is the energy needed to digest, absorb, and dispose of its nutrients, while gluconeogenesis is the production of glucose from fats or proteins.

Also, by eliminating foods on both Red lists, you're more likely to lose weight faster, since processed and sugary foods are associated with excess weight.

Finally, the lifestyle hacks mentioned above, such as intermittent fasting, can also contribute to weight loss, as it has been shown to increase metabolism and help burn more fat.

SUMMARY

The Banting diet may help you lose weight because it mixes a series of strategies that promote fat loss, such as increasing your feeling of fullness, eliminating processed and sugary foods, and practicing intermittent fasting.

Additional benefits

Following a LCHF diet like the Banting diet may lead to other potential health benefits.

Improved metabolic markers

LCHF diets may help reduce risk factors for both type 2 diabetes and heart disease.

Scientific evidence shows that they may reduce fasting insulin and blood sugar levels and improve insulin sensitivity, which is why LCHF diets are gaining popularity as potential first-line treatments for type 2 diabetes.

They also seem to decrease triglyceride and high blood pressure levels, increase HDL (good) cholesterol, and reverse nonalcoholic fatty liver disease.

For example, in one 12-week study in 26 people with excess weight, those following a

LCHF diet improved their glucose, insulin resistance, triglyceride, HDL (good) cholesterol, and HbA1c levels, compared with those in the HCLF group.

The HbA1c test — or glycated hemoglobin test — measures your average blood sugar levels over the past 3 months, and it's used as an evaluation tool for blood sugar control in people with diabetes.

Focuses on wholesome foods

By restricting processed and sugary foods, the diet almost automatically leads to a higher intake of wholesome, more nutritious foods.

High intakes of processed foods are associated with increased oxidative stress and inflammation, leading to the development of non-communicable chronic diseases (NCD) like cancer and heart disease and thus increasing the risk of mortality.

On the contrary, healthy eating patterns that focus on increasing fruit and vegetable intake seem to decrease the risk, as their nutrients help reduce oxidative stress and inflammation.

Thus, the Banting diet will most likely benefit your health.

SUMMARY

The Banting diet limits carbs and promotes the intake of wholesome foods, which leads to numerous health improvements.

Potential downsides

While the Banting diet offers numerous health benefits, its potential downsides cannot be ignored.

Highly restrictive

Aside from eliminating processed and sugary foods, the Banting diet's food lists also restrict grains and limit fruits, legumes, dairy, and nuts.

Evidence shows that consumption of those food groups may be beneficial for the prevention of type 2 diabetes, heart disease, and certain types of cancer.

Additionally, by restricting legumes, dairy, and nuts, and classifying tofu as a "gray area food," the diet makes it difficult for vegans and vegetarians to follow the plan.

Finally, the restrictive nature of the diet can make long-term maintenance difficult, which could end up hindering its effectiveness.

However, some may find that the support from online communities or the course's coaches and webinars is all they need to keep them going.

Long-term evidence is lacking

While the benefits of a LCHF eating pattern like the Banting diet seem promising, there's not enough human evidence to support its safety in the long run.

Some human and animal studies suggest potential adverse long-term effects of LCHF diets on LDL (bad) cholesterol levels and blood vessel elasticity, which may be detrimental to heart health.

However, more research is needed to understand how low carb diets affect heart health over longer time periods.

Therefore, some believe that the potential downsides of following this type of diet in the long term outweigh its potential benefits.

SUMMARY

The Banting diet restricts many food groups associated with multiple health benefits, and there's little evidence on its long-term health effects.

Sample menu

Here's what 3 days on the Banting diet would look like while following Phase 2 (Restoration phase):

Day 1

• Breakfast: 2–3 eggs — scrambled or fried — with avocado, cheese, tomato, and bacon; bulletproof coffee is also allowed

• Lunch: grilled fish fillet with sweet potato wedges and vegetable stir-fry

• Snack: Greek yogurt and macadamia nuts

• Dinner: a serving of protein of your choice — beef, pork, chicken, or fish — served with sautéed vegetables, a side salad, and cauliflower mash

Day 2

• Breakfast: 1/4 cup of Banting granola — toasted nuts and seeds with some spices — with yogurt and 1–2 hard-boiled eggs

• Lunch: a large grilled chicken salad with cottage cheese

• Snack: apple slices with nut butter

• Dinner: salmon fillet with avocado and grilled asparagus

Day 3

- Breakfast: coconut milk smoothie with mango, papaya, and a handful of nuts

- Lunch: beef fajitas with grilled onions, mushrooms, and peppers, and a side salad

- Snack: 1–2 cups (240–480 mL) of bone broth

- Dinner: pulled pork lettuce wraps with a side of roasted chickpeas

Although snacks are included, the program's advice is to avoid snacking and instead increase your previous meal's fat intake to curb hunger.

SUMMARY

The Banting diet encourages you to eat three LCHF meals and only snack if necessary.

The bottom line

The Banting diet is a type of low carb, high fat (LCHF) diet that mostly restricts starchy, processed, and sugary foods, instead promoting the intake of wholesome ones to lose weight rapidly.

Though there's no scientific evidence on the diet itself, studies on LCHF diets suggest that they may enhance metabolic markers for heart disease and diabetes.

Still, the diet is highly restrictive, and there's not enough evidence on the long-term effects of LCHF diets in humans.

Therefore, maintaining an intake of wholesome foods and reducing your intake of processed ones while shifting to a moderate-carb diet may be a more sustainable yet efficient weight loss approach.

A Low-Carb Meal Plan and Menu to Improve Your Health

A low-carb diet is a diet that restricts carbohydrates, such as those found in sugary foods, pasta and bread. It is high in protein, fat and healthy vegetables.

There are many different types of low-carb diets, and studies show that they can cause weight loss and improve health.

This is a detailed meal plan for a low-carb diet. It explains what to eat, what to avoid and includes a sample low-carb menu for one week.

Low-Carb Eating — The Basics

Your food choices depend on a few things, including how healthy you are, how much you exercise and how much weight you have to lose.

Consider this meal plan as a general guideline, not something written in stone.

Eat: Meat, fish, eggs, vegetables, fruit, nuts, seeds, high-fat dairy, fats, healthy oils and maybe even some tubers and non-gluten grains.

Don't eat: Sugar, HFCS, wheat, seed oils, trans fats, "diet" and low-fat products and highly processed foods.

Foods to Avoid

You should avoid these six food groups and nutrients, in order of importance:

• Sugar: Soft drinks, fruit juices, agave, candy, ice cream and many other products that contain added sugar.

• Refined grains: Wheat, rice, barley and rye, as well as bread, cereal and pasta.

• Trans fats: Hydrogenated or partially hydrogenated oils.

• Diet and low-fat products: Many dairy products, cereals or crackers are fat-reduced, but contain added sugar.

• Highly processed foods: If it looks like it was made in a factory, don't eat it.

• Starchy vegetables: It's best to limit starchy vegetables in your diet if you're following a very low-carb diet.

You must read ingredient lists even on foods labelled as health foods.

Low-Carb Food List — Foods to Eat

You should base your diet on these real, unprocessed, low-carb foods.

• Meat: Beef, lamb, pork, chicken and others; grass-fed is best.

- Fish: Salmon, trout, haddock and many others; wild-caught fish is best.

- Eggs: Omega-3-enriched or pastured eggs are best.

- Vegetables: Spinach, broccoli, cauliflower, carrots and many others.

- Fruits: Apples, oranges, pears, blueberries, strawberries.

- Nuts and seeds: Almonds, walnuts, sunflower seeds, etc.

- High-fat dairy: Cheese, butter, heavy cream, yogurt.

- Fats and oils: Coconut oil, butter, lard, olive oil and fish oil.

If you need to lose weight, be careful with cheese and nuts, as it's easy to overeat on them. Don't eat more than one piece of fruit per day.

Foods to Maybe Include

If you're healthy, active and don't need to lose weight, you can afford to eat a few more carbs.

- Tubers: Potatoes, sweet potatoes and some others.

• Unrefined grains: Brown rice, oats, quinoa and many others.

• Legumes: Lentils, black beans, pinto beans, etc. (if you can tolerate them).

What's more, you can have the following in moderation, if you want:

• Dark chocolate: Choose organic brands with at least 70% of cocoa.

• Wine: Choose dry wines with no added sugar or carbs.

Dark chocolate is high in antioxidants and may provide health benefits if you eat it in moderation. However, be aware that both dark chocolate and alcohol will hinder your progress if you eat/drink too much.

Beverages

• Coffee

• Tea

• Water

• Sugar-free carbonated beverages, like sparkling water.

A Sample Low-Carb Menu for One Week

This is a sample menu for one week on a low-carb diet plan.

It provides less than 50 grams of total carbs per day. However, if you're healthy and active you can eat slightly more carbs.

Monday

- Breakfast: Omelet with various vegetables, fried in butter or coconut oil.

- Lunch: Grass-fed yogurt with blueberries and a handful of almonds.

- Dinner: Bunless cheeseburger, served with vegetables and salsa sauce.

Tuesday

- Breakfast: Bacon and eggs.

• Lunch: Leftover burgers and veggies from the previous night.

• Dinner: Salmon with butter and vegetables.

Wednesday

• Breakfast: Eggs and vegetables, fried in butter or coconut oil.

• Lunch: Shrimp salad with some olive oil.

• Dinner: Grilled chicken with vegetables.

Thursday

• Breakfast: Omelet with various vegetables, fried in butter or coconut oil.

- Lunch: Smoothie with coconut milk, berries, almonds and protein powder.

- Dinner: Steak and veggies.

Friday

- Breakfast: Bacon and eggs.

- Lunch: Chicken salad with some olive oil.

- Dinner: Pork chops with vegetables.

Saturday

- Breakfast: Omelet with various veggies.

- Lunch: Grass-fed yogurt with berries, coconut flakes and a handful of walnuts.

- Dinner: Meatballs with vegetables.

Sunday

- Breakfast: Bacon and eggs.

- Lunch: Smoothie with coconut milk, a dash of heavy cream, chocolate-flavored protein powder and berries.

- Dinner: Grilled chicken wings with some raw spinach on the side.

Include plenty of low-carb vegetables in your diet. If your goal is to remain under 50 grams of carbs per day, there is room for plenty of veggies and one fruit per day.

Again, if you're healthy, lean and active, you can add some tubers like potatoes and sweet potatoes, as well as some healthy grains like oats.

Healthy, Low-Carb Snacks

There is no health reason to eat more than three meals per day, but if you get hungry between meals, here are some healthy, easy-to-prepare, low-carb snacks that can fill you up:

- A piece of fruit

- Full-fat yogurt

- One or two hard-boiled eggs

- Baby carrots

- Leftovers from the previous night

- A handful of nuts

- Some cheese and meat

Eating at Restaurants

At most restaurants, it's fairly easy to make your meals low-carb friendly.

1. Order a meat- or fish-based main dish.

2. Drink plain water instead of sugary soda or fruit juice.

3. Get extra vegetables instead of bread, potatoes or rice.

A Simple Low-Carb Shopping List

A good rule is to shop at the perimeter of the store, where the whole foods are more likely to be found.

Focusing on whole foods will make your diet a thousand times better than the standard Western diet.

Organic and grass-fed foods are also popular choices and often considered healthier, but they're typically more expensive.

Try to choose the least processed option that still fits into your price range.

- Meat (beef, lamb, pork, chicken, bacon)

- Fish (fatty fish like salmon is best)

- Eggs (choose omega-3 enriched or pastured eggs if you can)

- Butter

- Coconut oil

- Lard

- Olive oil

- Cheese

- Heavy cream

- Sour cream

- Yogurt (full-fat, unsweetened)

- Blueberries (fresh or frozen)

- Nuts

- Olives

- Fresh vegetables (greens, peppers, onions, etc.)

- Frozen vegetables (broccoli, carrots, various mixes)

- Condiments (sea salt, pepper, garlic, mustard, etc.)

Clear your pantry of all unhealthy temptations if you can, such as chips, candy, ice cream, sodas, juices, breads, cereals and baking ingredients like refined flour and sugar.

The Bottom Line

Low-carb diets restrict carbs, such as those found in sugary and processed foods, pasta and bread. They're high in protein, fat and healthy vegetables.

Studies show that they can cause weight loss and improve health.

The above meal plan gives you the basics of healthy, low-carb eating.

If you need a comprehensive list of low-carb

recipes that are both simple and delicious,

check out this article on